My Spiritual Journey with HIV

Mary F. Moreno

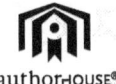

Bloomington, IN   Milton Keynes, UK

authorHOUSE®

AuthorHouse™
1663 Liberty Drive, Suite 200
Bloomington, IN 47403
www.authorhouse.com
Phone: 1-800-839-8640

First published by AuthorHouse 11/20/2007

ISBN: 978-1-4343-0213-7 (sc)

Printed in the United States of America
Bloomington, Indiana

This book is printed on acid-free paper.

CONTENTS

FORWARD

J can remember the time very vividly, just over 21 years ago. I was a young man, married with three boys, and my Mom told me about her news she received from the hospital. Her recent operation required a blood transfusion, and some of the blood she received was tainted with the HIV virus, and now she had a positive HIV status. 'What did that mean?' Those words seem foreign to me, for at the time, this virus was rarely found in heterosexual women. At that time, Mom was upset and felt victimized.

"*She* did her research and educated us all on how the virus could not be passed along to one of us. She wanted to put us at ease, so that we could continue as we were and more importantly, so that we wouldn't do or say anything to upset my younger 10 year old sister, Anita. She insisted that she was still going to be a functional part of our lives as a mother and wife. She assured us that she could still show affection towards us with embraces and kisses, which all of her 5 children and husband certainly still needed from her. She was determined not to let her infection bring her down. She believed, more strongly than ever, that she deserved to live a normal life and boy, let me tell you, (no virus was going to get in her way).

When we were young, my siblings and I put up with…a lot of restaurant dramas..knowing that this is a woman you want on your side. She will fight for her rights as a human being, a citizen, a minority woman, and as an…employee. After weeks of court hearings and out of court meetings, she won this battle, and in the process she made history…

"Throughout the trial period, my mom kept her faith that she would prevail. Anyone who has met her knows how deeply rooted her faith in God is. It has become a cornerstone in her life and she has passed this onto her children.

Whenever she found out that me, or one of my loved ones were in need, she would light a candle and say a prayer on our behalf. She believes that Christ Spirit within her above all else has allowed her to rise above the obstacles she has come across. I believe this too, as I am a witness to it. ...if you were to see her..., you might see an elderly, graying, hobbling woman that may appear timid and vulnerable, but do not under estimate her. She is worthy of your attention, as she is a living example of determination and spirit. She is 'What moves Me.'

"*Ladies* and Gentleman, at this time, I would like to introduce to you, Mary Moreno, my mentor, my motivator, and my mom."

(The above speech is in part one given by our oldest son, Roger I. Moreno, Sr. at the pre-ceremonies for the AIDS Ride for Life in 1995.)

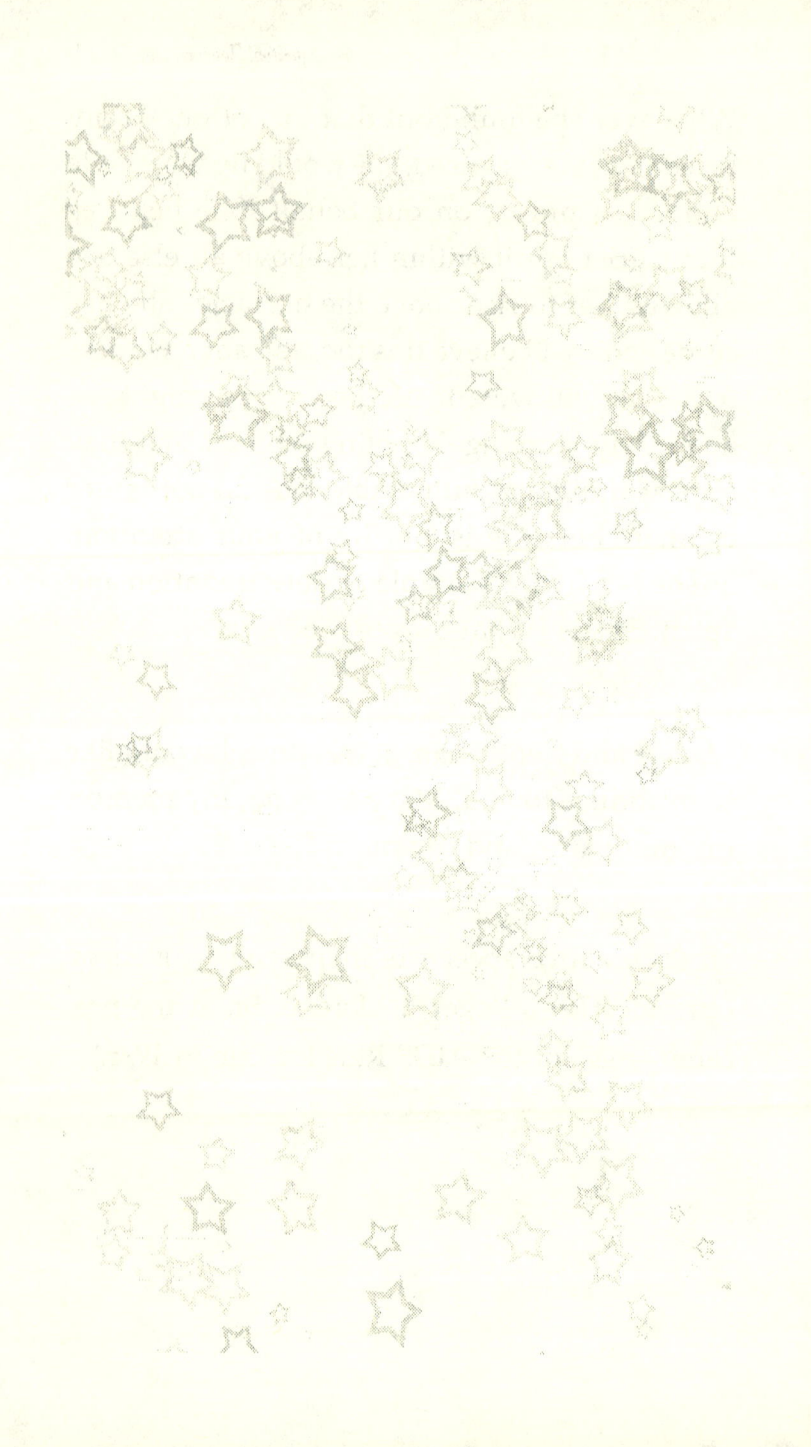

My Spiritual
Journey With HIV

While listening to the March rain this early morning of 2006, as I've done numerous times over the years, I became focused on the events in my life since learning I was infected with the virus called HIV. I remember a day at work in November of 1987. I received a telephone call from my then GYN. He spoke to me directly, which was unusual; usually I would receive calls from his office staff reminding me of the need to schedule an annual checkup. This call was quite different. He began by telling me a national federal program called "Project Lookback" had contacted him to advise him one of his patients may have contacted HIV from a blood transfusion; and I was that person. Naturally, I went into a state of shock as I was told I needed to be tested ASAP. He continued by telling me I needed to go to a local hospital to be tested; arrangements were set up with the lab there and only two staff persons were aware of my coming. It was all very hush-hush and secretive.

Tears were flowing from my eyes as I hung up the phone and proceeded to dial the phone to contact my best friend and soul mate, my husband (Gabby) of 27 years at that time. I closed the door to my office and somehow managed to tell Gabby what I had just learned. Later, after I got home after work, Gabby and I tearfully talked about the news I was given earlier and the implications on our lives and the lives of our five children and other family members. We were both in a high state of shock.

Our lives in 1987 had already experienced major events. One was happy and exciting: I was the first one in my family to earn a masters degree; it fulfilled a dream my father had all his life; however, the timing was such I decided not to attend the graduation and all its grandeur.

Another major event was the death of Gabby's mom (Mo), who lived with us for 25 years and suffered the last eleven of these years with colon cancer. She died the last day of May 1987, and we were still grieving for her. It seemed like we were experiencing one of the darkest times of our married life. At that time, I believed I had received an early death sentence, and wondered how were we going to cope.

That evening, Gabby and I began discussing critical issues regarding the news we received that eventful day: like which members of our families were we going to tell, especially our immediate ones. We decided we would tell the older four children, but not our youngest, Anita; she was only 10 years old and the death of Mo hit her especially hard. Not only her youth affected how Anita felt about Mo's death, but also the fact Anita and Mo always had a very close relationship. Anita was also very close to her next sibling, Loretta, who although 11 years older, has always been like a "second" mother to her younger sister. At the time I believe this was a great asset for Anita; she leaned more toward Loretta for comfort and understanding, especially during the last few days of Mo's life. With the help of the wonderful people of Hospice, we were able to allow Mo to die in dignity, here at our home on her favorite couch in our living room. We invited Mo's other children and grandchildren to be with her and us during her last days. During these days, it felt like we had a celebration of Mo's life, allowing everyone to talk about incidents we had experienced: often we laughed during our recollections, at other times, we could only cry and hug each other. It was not only a tribute to Mo, but we were able to voice how she had affected our lives all these years we lived together. I will always be grateful to God and our families for allowing this time for us to share these special moments with each other and with our beloved Mo.

It wasn't until Anita was 14 years old or so that Gabby and I decided we could tell her about the disease I was infected with; her only comment was, "Why didn't you tell me sooner?" I had no good answer for her. At the time, Anita was working on a school project. She had to select and write a short article about someone she admired. Ironically, Anita decided to write about Ryan White, a young man who lived with and died of AIDS. A few years after his death, federal funding for combating the disease was enacted and named the Ryan White Care Act. I remember thinking how God works in mysterious ways! To this day, I am in awe of the way God intervened and assisted Gabby and me in our struggle to decided when and how we would tell our youngest family member this profound health information.

I now feel strongly my life with HIV was in answer to my then prayers for help in learning to grow closer to our Almighty. And although the time between 1987 and August 1990 was a time of denial for me about my HIV status, I tend to believe it was a grieving process God allowed me to go through. I remember during August 3-5, 1990, I was attending a local training session provided by the employee union I held membership in at the time; it was on HIV in the workplace. I was in the women's restroom and encountered the trainer, Janeice Fogg, who was a member of the National AFCIO organization, going around the country educating members of different employee unions on both health and legal issues involved with this horrible disease. As we talked in the restroom, it was the first time I felt comfortable enough to disclose my HIV status to anyone outside of family and a few close friends. Janeice immediately told me part of the training involved having someone living with the virus speak at the end; further, that the person designated for this training was too ill to attend and asked if I would tell my story. I was immediately taken aback by her request, and told Janeice I had never spoken publicly about my status. I expressed my concern of how going public would affect our youngest child, Anita, in view of the fact the training was being video taped. Janeice assured me they would not tape the session if I chose to participate. That turned out to be my first experience as an HIV/AIDS educator. At the time, I had no inkling how emotional telling my story would turn out. Expressing all the feelings I had kept inside all those three or so years seemed to me like one of the volcanoes erupting I had helped Anita type about in one of her earlier school reports. Later and quiet naturally, tears overflowed as I drove home from the training. It was like the floodgates of my anger, sorrow and depression were released all at one time, and I began to live like I wasn't on a path towards death. This was the beginning of a new career for me, based on my personal journey with a new lifelong partner called HIV.

As an A-type personality, I began keeping a journal-type record of my HIV talks. I went so far as making a list of all the events and places I spoke at, including dates, the event and purpose of my talks and the number or estimate of participants in attendance at each event. As of March 2006, I have compiled a 13 page list in thirteen 2-3 inch binders which also include pictures and printed speeches I have written for each event, some being duplicates of previous talks. The special parts of each of these events are the pictures I've taken with new and old friends I've made throughout these years. Some have died since our encounters, others are still around keeping in touch through e-mails and personal contacts while attending conferences/events we have been present at the same time. Recently, as I was reviewing the list, I began recalling particular incidents of many of these events, some of which are detailed in the following pages.

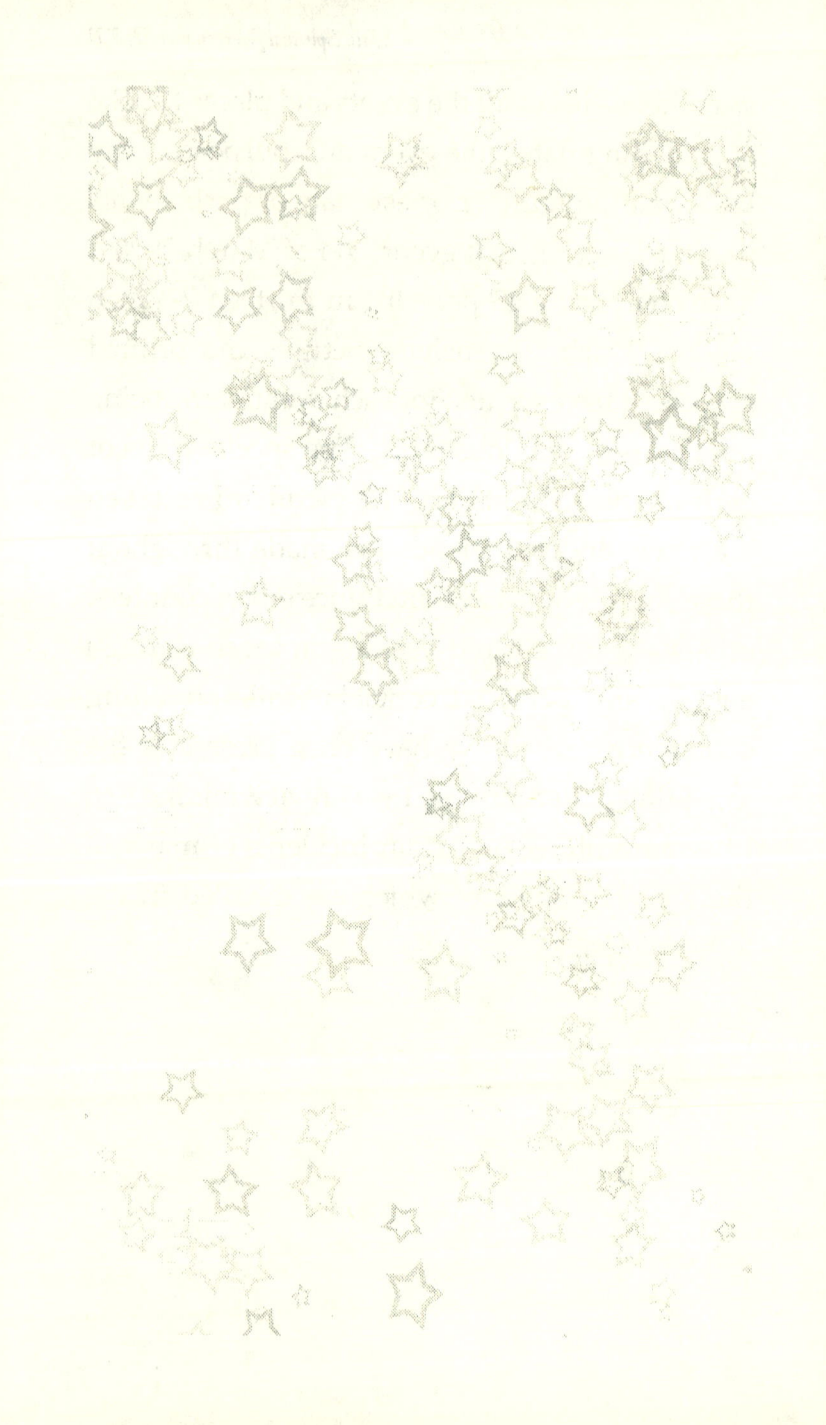

GETTING MY FEET WET

As I think about this initial public talk about how my life was changing since knowing of my HIV+ status, it seems odd a high-profile pharmaceutical company financially supported the workshop. The workshop focused on early initiation of anti-viral therapy for health care and social/medical workers. I spoke how the stress at my work led me to begin seeing a local female psychologist. I described her as fantastic: sensitive, understanding woman who took the time to listen to my needs. We discussed issues involved with the stress of my job, and my need to locate a women's support group to deal with the stress, which, at the time, was non-existent. The psychologist directed me to a local Center for Attitudinal Healing, where I "fell" into the Adult Healing Group for persons dealing with all kinds of catastrophic illnesses. There at the

Center I became familiar with many different techniques of relaxation, meditation and positive mind thinking by focusing each week on 1 of 12 Principles of Attitudinal Healing. I attended these weekly sessions for almost six months. Up until the last month, I was the only person (and female) dealing with HIV. There was an HIV group that met there every Friday, but all were males. At that time, I had a mental block, hate, whatever with HIV/AIDS males. I believed that as most were gay, they were responsible for my contacting this virus. It took a long time, but I eventually realized everyone dealing with this catastrophic illness needed understanding, compassion and most importantly, L O V E.

Up until this time, I was in denial of the need to deal with my HIV status, and a new goal evolved for me. I realized I needed to find a medical practitioner that above all would take the time to educate me about my disease, listen to my needs (especially as a female), and perhaps help me find a female support group. At that time I did not consider myself as a female activist; however, for over a year I experienced changes in my body. I instinctively knew something was wrong, and being in the dark as to what to expect with my illness. I was afraid to contact my then male physician to ask questions about things such as having a yeast infection for almost a month, frequent pain in my glands under my arms which would disappear or move to another area, my tongue turning white for a day, off and on, and finally, fever blisters on my mouth when I didn't even have a cold. Sometimes, I could barely swallow water.

I never knew that the normal count/marker for my body's immune system should be between 800-1200, and an abnormal count begins at 500 and lower. As discussed above, when I attended the employee union AIDS training in August 1990, my education in AIDS began. Soon after this training, I went to the largest AIDS agency in town and began counseling with their education coordinator, Sylvia Lopez. Sylvia introduced me to nutrition education as well as general education and suggested appropriate reference materials.

While at this AIDS agency, I became aware of a newly formed female support group in South Austin, coordinated by another social worker, Barbara. In October 1990, we began as a 7-member group meeting weekly. After a year, we were down to 5 members. Since then, I have repeatedly realized that l learned more about my disease in the last 3 months of 1990, than I had over the 3 years since I learned of my diagnosis. Some of the women in that group were gay and exchanged a lot of information on how they addressed HIV/ AIDS related illnesses, sexuality, how and when to tell your child (ren) about your health status, to name a few.

I also found a female physician, Dr Paula Rogge. At that first visit, she gave me a two-sided folder filled with educational material which helped me better understand the meaning of my diagnosis and things to expect in the future. She referred me for other diagnostic exams, including a mammogram.

I began to realize I was and to this date still am a statistic==a good one at that. When I chose to relate my experience with HIV at the August 1990 workshop, people were amazed at my longevity with this disease, even though it was a short six-year period. At that time people were dying within as short a time as six months of diagnosis and as long as 2-3 years. I was asked specifically what I had done to stay so well after 6 years. I told them it was a renewed faith that began two weeks after receiving that fateful blood transfusion during a major surgery in February 1984, and also my new desire to become more educated about this new, additional life-long partner called HIV.

I have spoken at many, many conferences and other venues of my spiritual reawakening while recuperating from major surgery early in 1984. I remember my mother one morning coming into my bedroom with a few new magazines. I realized I was tired of reading, and TV no longer interested me. I had been in bed for almost two weeks and I was anxious to become active. Suddenly I got out of bed and reached over to my desk and picked up the family bible given by our local Catholic church. Flipping through the book, I stopped on a page and realized it was the beginning of the Book of Job. I read the story several times and began to see similar incidents to my life at that time. I realized I was not the spiritual and good-hearted person as was Job. But after years of trying to be a good person, I could not understand what I had done to deserve so many trials at this time in my life. I must admit it took me years to more clearly realize it was God's way of answering a request

I had made several years earlier: to find ways to grow closer to Him. It was also a reminder of the saying "Be careful what you pray for as you will receive an answer, but it may not be as you would expect."

In August 1991, I submitted a comprehensive 7-page written proposal entitled, "an HIV Pilot Project" addressed to the then City Manager. The project proposed an integrated comprehensive HIV educational component and support services for employees and their families. HIV education to all employees at all levels would be developed and a designated liaison would assist in directing those with HIV/AIDS in need to social services provided within the community. Possible funding sources were outlined. It was; however, disappointing that the City Manager showed no interest in the proposal, which led me to believe she was either ignorant of the need and/or just not interested to pursue a program on this sensitive issue.

Gabby and I attended the First Western Regional Conference on Women and HIV the latter part of October 1991, held outside of San Diego, CA, in La Hoya. It gave me new hope and I gained new friendships such as Carole

Norman, a nurse first as well as an HIV/AIDS educator and coordinator of this conference. We became instant friends, and have remained close even with the distance between us. Carole took a special interest in Gabby, and me and over the years since our first encounter, we remain close through e-mails and correspondence. Carol and her husband, Roy, have visited us here at our home, as we visited them at each subsequent conference held every 2 years thereafter. The conference covered a wide range of topics I had not heard before; quite naturally it was a huge learning experience for me, and I took copious notes. During the conference I met an AIDS activist who lived in Oakland, Rebecca Dennison. She had just organized an HIV/AIDS women's group called WORLD (Women Organized to Respond to Life-threatening Diseases). Rebecca was infected with the virus as I. We spoke briefly at that time; we would become close friends beginning at a later date.

The next year, early spring of 1992, I did what many believed was the "unthinkable" but brave undertaken. I came "out" with my HIV status in the March 1992 issue of a nationwide magazine,

Public Employee in an article called, "An AFSCME Grandmother Faces AIDS." The author, Fred J. Solowey, would later receive an award for his article; I would lose my job later in May of that year.

What followed were attempts to get me to quit: my computer was taken away from my work area at the same time I was assigned to compile an end of the year federal report in a very short turnaround timeframe. Additionally, I had no training in the preparation of this extensive and complex report, and a person with more than 12 years of experience and training had let the report sit on her desk for almost 2 months. Via telephone, with the help from federal oversight employees in another city, I was able to not only compile and write the report, but later these federal staff told me the report was on time and the best one received from our office in 15 years. I was only able to complete the report by using my time on a home computer evenings and weekends. I, however, received no comments regarding the report from my superiors, one way or the other. Often times and without notice, I would be moved to another part of the area. In addition, work assignments were not at the caliber or level I had done prior to the "outing" of my HIV status.

It was during this time period, I began going to counseling session with a Catholic priest at our church. After a few sessions, the advice my priest gave me was for me to start praying for the manager who was giving me the most grief. I was so glad the priest could not read my thoughts: "What, you want me to pray for that B…. M……F…!" A few days later, I thought about the priest's advice, but I did nothing at that time. Some time passed and again I remembered what the priest had said; I guess I must have been feeling charitable at the time as I began to pray the Hail Mary. At first it was just rote, I just said the words with no feelings. Months later as I was praying, I realized I was the one being affected; anger and frustration began to subside. No, I did not begin to feel any love for the man, just neutral thoughts and feelings. A long time later I was able to forgive and let go of the anger and hate. But now back to my work experiences.

More harassment continued towards me. I remember I became ill, and asked to take sick leave in order to contact Dr. Rogge. My request was denied, so I called my union representative (rep). She, however, was at another office helping another employee save their job. The union steward in our building also tried to help, but he was denied as well. My union rep sent over her secretary to sit with me until she (the rep) could come to help me. I was sitting there with the secretary, tears rolling down my face, and softly saying over and over, "God, why have you forsaken me?" Finally, my union rep arrived, spoke to the person in charge and within a few minutes was able to obtain approval for me to take sick leave.

The last major incident occurred early in April 1992. As noted earlier in my story, already experiencing some health problems associated with the virus, the increased job stress along with direct harassment actions taken by my place of employment after the magazine article became public, only served to the demise of my overall health. I remember arriving to work on a Monday early in April 1992. I had been ill all weekend, and as I arrived at my desk I placed a call to Dr. Rogge to let her know about my illness: a hurtful yeast infection and herpes in my mouth so painful, I could not eat or drink a thing. I left a message with the doctor's nurse and asked for a return call from the doctor. Immediately after I hung up the phone, my immediate supervisor called me into his office and began discussing a new assignment, a major research project which required training and experience, none of which I had the opportunity to acquire. I told the supervisor of my weekend health problems and was awaiting a call back from my doctor. He went on discussing the assignment; he ignored my concern of the lack of training and experience to complete the assignment in a thorough and knowledgeable manner.

My phone rang at my desk and as I approached to take the call, the supervisor was right behind me as I spoke to Dr. Rogge. I was totally embarrassed to have to discuss sensitive female health problems within earshot of the supervisor, but he would not move away. He did, however, approve my taking sick leave to go to the doctor's office. As it turned out, Dr. Rogge ordered me to bed rest for the rest of the week, along with a few new prescriptions. When I returned to work I was surprised my bosses said nothing of my absence.

Instead, a month or so passed. Then one day I was told to go up to another floor and meet with personnel staff and my immediate boss. I responded I would go only if my union repr would be able to be present. At the set time, my rep and I met with personnel staff and my boss. I was handed a letter, which stated in part I did not go home the month before due to illness; instead, it was because I did not want to complete an assignment given to me that day, and if it happen again, I would be fired. Again, the new assignment required completing a major review report and again, I had neither experience nor training to complete this complex work.

As often happens in these instances, the above incident happen on a Friday. Over the weekend, Gabby and I talked extensively about my work situation. When I cried out, "I have a right to keep my job and work and keep my health insurance." To which my husband responded, "Would you rather be right or be dead?" I thought about what he said for a long time; we then made the decision I would resign and then take action to correct the injustice. In May 1992, I lost my job; however, it was not the first time I had taken on an activist role regarding employment. I won a federal EEO case back in the 1970s; however, that's another story for another time.

Later that summer, Gabby and I decided to invite my parents for a trip to New Orleans. I remembered my mother (who lived in San Antonio) telling me she always wanted to go to New Orleans, but for reasons I won't go into here, she never went. I called them up; when my Dad answered, I jokingly told him, "Gabby and I plan to make a trip to New Orleans and we want to invite Mamo. You can go too, if you promise to behave.

As it turned out, we took them, our youngest, Anita, and her "twin" cousin, Noelle (one month older than Anita), who also lived in San Antonio. We located a motel with a huge corner room. It was perfect for us. Of all of us, my Mom (Mamo) was having the most fun. She loved to shop at Woolworth's, so we stop at each one, 3 blocks between each of them. We shopped and shopped, and shopped again. My father, bless his heart, got stressed out with all our stops to shop, but he was cool. Then the rains came! But we still needed to go to the famous "Pat O'Brien" pub. I laugh now as we had Mamo and Pampo go unto the place, sit in the rain at a table while I took a photo of them drinking a glass of something. Poor Gabby stood outside in the rain, with Anita and Noelle as they were underage and not allowed to enter.

Anita and Noelle loved the trip. They made friends with the motel cook, and he would bake them fresh cookies each night and let them into the pool to swim.

As I anticipated, when we returned from our trip, I would not be able to get another job. I also started experiencing more health problems and needed more medications whose costs required my going for assistance at the largest local AIDS agency. My mother came from San Antonio and went with me to sign up for Medicare with the help of an assigned caseworker, Becky. I considered Becky as my guardian angel. At 4 ft.11inches or so, she was a force who could accomplish so much. Becky and I became close friends beyond her role as my caseworker, plus she makes the best potato salad in town!

To keep busy that summer, I began organizing my home. First, I went through 30 boxes of my 5 kids school papers and reduced them to a few

8x11 boxes per child. It was a real challenge, as being a pack rat by nature; I saved almost every piece. By the time I finished, I threw away around 30 large trash bags

We then invited Mary Bo and John Gil (Gabby always called him JOHNNY Gil, Jr.), our best friends to take a trip to the Balloon Fest, October 8-12, 1992. We also took my parents (Mamo) and (Pampo). We drove up there in our 1992 Van. Johnny drove us to and from Albuquerque; however, we stayed in a 2-story rented hotel in Santa Fe. It was a great trip, restful as well as full of sites to see in both cities. When all the balloons ascending into the sky, it was awesome! And of course, we did a lot of shopping, especially my Mamo. She was one of those people who could "shop until she dropped." She never bought much, but boy did she like to look at EVERYTHING! It would drive my father crazy. But as she was with me, he knew better than complain; I would read him the right act or should I say, the "Moreno" right act.

Mary (Bo) and Johnny are excellent companions for a road trip; always agreeable, laughing and having fun. We had been on many vacations along with our kids and their kids. At Mary's request, we stopped at a place called Loretto Miraculous Chapel. The chapel was very small, holds about 20 people and hanging all around the walls of a smaller room, which looked like it was an addition to the chapel, were crutches and other memorabilia. Feelings of peace and serenity surrounded me and it felt like a big weight was lifted from my shoulders.

We all knelt down in a pew and prayed. Mary Bo, who was kneeling next to Gabby leaned over and whispered, "Maybe we'd better not pray too long for you wife; otherwise, she might outlive us all." Everyone was laughing so hard; we all got up and left the chapel.

Ironically, I did outlive Mary Bo; at that time she was in remission from breast cancer. She died on December 26, 2003.

Then in early fall of that year, another infected woman in our support group I described earlier, Odile, and I started a spiritual support group at one of our local catholic church. As it turned out, usually Odile and I were the only two in attendance along with the priest. It was sad to realize the lack of interest for spirituality guidance. No amount of placing information in church bulletins all over town seemed to help. Odile died of AIDS related illnesses the following year, and I missed her for a long time thereafter. And, of course, the support group was no longer

As I stated earlier, after resigning from my job in May 1992, and not able to find another job, I became an outspoken activist on HIV/AIDS. In January 1993, the Austin Business Journal wrote an article called "Working with AIDS, a business matter," with my picture on the front page. The article not only spoke of my treatment at my last employment, but also on the nationwide need for employers to become educated about the disease and to develop "reasonable accommodations" for all its employees infected, which I believed was not done in my situation. I was able to prove that "BUT FOR the fact I was infected with HIV, my employee union after 2 years was unable to transfer me to another department wherein they had formerly moved employees from the "blue collar" category to department heads. Further, the timeframe for this action occurred in as short a time as 30 minutes to the longest of 30 days.

The next month, February 1993, a well-known panel member of the National Commission of AIDS, Mary Fisher, a 44-year old artist from Florida, gave a formidable speech. Ms. Fisher was known for an emotional speech she gave a year earlier in Houston at the Republican National Convention. On Feb. 2, 1993, I was able to speak with Ms. Fisher briefly. She inspired me to continue with my new work as an HIV/AIDS educator.

One of the most memorable times of that year was a road trip we made during Spring Break, March 15-21, 1993. My parents (Mamo and Pampo), our oldest son, Roger, and two of his sons, Joshua and Stephen, along with our youngest, Anita, all squeezed into our 1992 van for the trip. I loved the fact we were a four generational family on this trip. As we got closer to D.C., it was snowing and we were redirected off the main highway and ended up somewhere in Virginia. We found a motel and by this time it was around 2:a.m. The desk clerk told us his night staff was unable to drive to the motel and we would have to make up our own beds. Not a problem;

Around 7a.m. or so, I was awakened by loud laughter outside. Half asleep, I went to a window, looked out and was surprised to see Roger and his sons having a snowball fight. They were having a blast! I realized I desperately needed a cup of coffee.

We then drove into D.C. and did the usual tourist things. Once, while we were in line to enter the Capitol, I heard Roger tell his sons, "You guys are going to look awfully funny doing push-ups in front of the capitol. He then saved the day for all; he took his sons and Anita, headed back to our hotel, had his sons write a 50-pg. report why they should not behave as they did, and later took them and Anita to the zoo!

From February 1993 until the fall of 1994, I presented around 35 or so HIV/AIDS presentations to schools, U.T. students (one-on-one), councils, Hispanic groups and once to the National AFl-CIO conference in Washington, D.C. I was also appointed by local mayor to serve on the HIV Planning Council. This group is responsible for making allocations of federal and local dollars for HIV/AIDS services in our city, and several surrounding counties; in addition, I was voted the first Co-Chair of the Planning Council.

The highlight of that year was when I received notice of a scholarship awarded by NAPWA (the

National Association of People With AIDS/HIV) to attend the 10th International HIV Conference in Yokahama, Japan. I was ecstatic; unfortunately, my husband was not able to go with me.

Another woman awarded a scholarship to Japan was Rebecca Dennison from Oakland, California, whom I had met at the first Western Regional HIV and Women conference, September 1991. At this conference, Rebecca and I had time for a nice visit, exchanging info and what we were doing. I told her another social worker and I was co-founding a women's HIV group here in Austin. And when I told her we were trying to put together a 3-day retreat similar to the one Rebecca had in place with her group, she offered to help us out. We exchanged e-mail and phone numbers. Upon returning to Austin, I passed the information on to co-founder Sylvia Lopez.

With the help of Rebecca Dennison of WORLD in California, Sylvia Lopez and I co-founded the first Central Texas women's groups, which became WOMEN RISING. We planned and held our first 3-day retreat in April 1995, with Rebecca as one of the presenters. We would expand our program to include a weekly support group, one-day retreats, as well as an intense HIV University. I was in the first class; we planned our curriculum, selected "deans" as leaders of different parts of the university and attended classes. We also received a diploma and held a graduation party at the completion of the university.

I had met and made so many new friends at Yokahama. And even though our youngest child asked me to bring her a China doll, they were out of my price range, so I took a picture of one and brought it to Anita. Before I went on this trip, I was very concerned how those of us infected would be treated in Japan, especially since I read earlier that doctors there did not seem eager to take care of us if we became ill. I realized later, I had nothing to fear. The Japanese people were so warm and caring, and made my stay there so memorable. The food I could take it or leave it, mostly leave it, but everything else was fantastic. Even though we were on scholarships, we stayed at one of the most luxury hotels, we were served warm meals at lunch and even a special reception was held for us. I even got to meet and picture taken with the Japanese AIDS poster boy, Toshihiro Oishi, then a 25 year old PWA (People with HIVAIDS). He was one of about 3,000 infected attendees, with approximately 10,000 total people attending the six-day conference.

As I look at all the pictures I took of my friends, my only regret is that I failed to write their names on the picture upon returning, and with my memory not as good as then, I only recognized a couple of them: Marlene Diaz of New York and Sharon Lund. The last time I spoke to Marlene was right after September 11th. She was just a few blocks away from the towers, and she had a hard time verifying her young daughter was okay at school. Days later, Marlene let me know she and daughter were fine. Sharon I haven't spoken to in a while, but my e-mails to her have not been returned, so I assume she's okay. Both of these women are strong advocates and very active in HIV.

The AIDS quilts on display at the conference were so colorful and awesome; they came from all over the world. One of the fun things I did was attend a flower-making/design workshop; it was so cool, but I doubt I could design a flower arrangement today. I brought home a pretty pair of lavender (Anita's favorite color in the purple family) pj's for Anita, who to this day wears them. My mom loved a black lace fan I gave her upon returning from Japan, which Gabby and I passed on to our granddaughter Rachel after my mom died in 1995. Dad's gift of a set of Chinese massages balls may still be at his home. All in all, this is one trip I'll always remember, I hope!

Returning from Japan, I then had to face a two-week trial of court case I filed against my former employer. When I first started this process, I had no idea how long it would take. Two years earlier (almost to the same month) I went to San Antonio, and filed a grievance at the federal court there, along with a notebook containing 75 documents I collected to verify my claim. As it turned out, the woman who got my case was new, never had a case before. Of course I got nervous when I learned of this; sure enough, after four or so months I received a notice from them that denied my claim. I was very disappointed; I believed the evidence I had was more than sufficient to make my case. Later, I realized my way was not in God's plan.

I didn't give up, and I don't recall how, but I found an attorney who would take my case; he was a Godsend, literally. Very knowledgeable in

EEO law, he and his partner began reviewing my 75 documents, and after numerous meetings to review and ask me questions, they determined I had a good case. My best recollection of the trial itself is I became very aware of God's presence throughout the trial: first, the judge was known as one of the fairest in our county; his wife, also an attorney, worked pro bono for the AIDS agency I was hooked up with. Family and friends were very supportive, and I was always calm throughout the trial even though some of the witnesses lied through their teeth, some even had been my friends for over 12 years. The best thing is my husband, Gabby, was by my side each and every day, always lifting my spirits when I needed, and making me laugh with his funny ways. I still tell him he's "The Wind Beneath my Wings."

Towards the end of the trial, my lawyers would tell me even if I didn't win the case, I had won in that I opened people's minds to what a PWA may face when people find out they are infected. I never thought about whether I would or would not win the case; I had already placed my faith in God and awaited His decision. At the beginning of the trial, our local paper's headline was "Ex

...worker tells of harassment." Seven days later, it read: "Woman with HIV wins suit against...." What most people were unaware of is the stress I went through after the jury ruled in my favor. The judge put both sides in mediation; that's because the defendants advised they intended to appeal the decision. I remember telling my husband, "They think they can outlive me, but I'll show them!" It took more than two weeks to go through this process; when the mediator saw how stressed out I had become, he told me something I believed came from my Maker, "Ms Moreno, there is no amount of money that can compensate you for all you've gone through, but..."

Even though I got only 1/3 of the original amount awarded by the jury and I did not get my job back, I believed I had won. I forced my former employer to realize they would be held responsible for not treating people living with this virus the respect and fairness everyone deserves. At that time I really believed I had made a difference. A few years later, I realized not so. I met a young woman who had just joined Women Rising; she had just quit her job at the same employment and on almost under the same circumstances. She chose not to pursue legal action, as she had no family in town; instead, she quit her job and moved to Florida to live with her only living relative, a brother and his wife. I've never heard from her again. I just keep her in my prayers.

STEPPING STONES
IN A NEW CAREER

As I was watching the Holy Mass on TV today, May 7, 2006, I was impressed by the whole 2-hour ceremony. The commentary explained the meaning of the songs sung by the choir, which states, "Where there is God, there is love." The words struck my heart remembering the words of many of my infected sisters I met while attending local, statewide and national HIV/AIDS conferences. Although they spoke in different words, each told of the same disheartened experience of being literally thrown out of their home by their families. As I began my journey living with this disease, I cried every time one of these brave souls told their story. Even today, I believe this type of treatment is still true. Some of the women had their child(ren) ripped away from them by family who thought they were doing the "right" thing. I'm not one to judge myself, but I have experience part of this hurt during my personal journey, which happen around 1996. That's a story for a later chapter.

My first national conference occurred Jan 18-24, 1995. I served as a panelist at the National Labor Leaders' Conference on Women & HIV, held in Washington, D.C, sponsored by the Center for Disease Control (CDC) and the Coalition of Labor Union Women. This was the first time I heard an infected woman talk about her experience as described in a previous paragraph; her mother took away her daughter and put her own daughter (the speaker) out on the streets. The positive part of that trip was our oldest daughter, Eunice, joined us for a couple of days. We all toured D.C. and even spent a day at the National Zoo, along with the usual visit to Union Station, among other sites,

The following month, I attended a 4-day HIV Infection in Women Conference, "Setting a new Agenda," February 22-24, 1995, again in D.C. I attended on a scholarship, and my roommate whom I met at the International Conference on

AIDS, Marlene Diaz, and I had the opportunity to really bond and become close friends. At this time, however, I have not heard from Marlene since I spoke to her right after 9/11.

The latter part of our visit was with Janeice Fogg, my new friend whom I met in 1990. Sadly, however, it was during this visit with Janeice I received a long-distance call from family members in San Antonio, TX. My mother became very ill and was in the hospital.

As I was already schedule to fly back home the next day, I did so, repacked, and Gabby and I drove to San Antonio. For two weeks, we spent every day at the hospital along with my 2 sisters and brother. I kept hoping and praying my mother (we called "Mamo") would get well and walk out of that hospital. She never did. One day while at the hospital, I received a long distance call from our youngest daughter, Anita, who was in tears; she spoke about the harassment she was experiencing at her high school trip with the dance team. It seemed the director was giving Anita a hard time about her boyfriend following them in his car on their bus trip. I immediately put on my "activist" hat; talked to Anita until she calmed down, and told her I would speak to the school principal upon our return.

My mother's passing on March 15, 1995, was horrific for my siblings and me. On her last day, I had all family members and close friends at the hospital that day to come into her room while we prayed the rosary for her. I also had each person talk about her and tell how she had impacted their life. I believe it was a beautiful tribute to my mother, who all her life as mother, co-owner of Dad's dry cleaners and wife, was a "rock" to our family, especially in her quiet and painful endurance of hard work and marital struggles.

A few days after returning from my mother's funeral, I contacted the high school principal I spoke of above and made an appointment. Once there, I gave him an earful of how I believed Anita's dance director was wrong in that I knew of other instances wherein other girls were allowed to have their boyfriends do the same thing as Anita's boyfriend at that time. Oddly the principal (an African American) talked about similar incidents occurring in the past with this dance director. He assured me he would speak to the dance director. I say oddly because if he spoke to this director, nothing came of it. Eventually the Director resigned a few years later, but I was very disappointed as to my knowledge, she was neither fired nor even reprimanded

Between February and August of that year I continued to make presentations locally and statewide. I was even interviewed (for the first time) by Nathan Linsk, PhD., of Chicago's AIDS Training & Education Center. The topic was on HIV in Older Adults. Nathan was founder of the HIV over Fifty (NAHOF) which he asked me to join, and I did.

Both my husband, Gabby, and I served as panelists at the 3rd Western Regional HIV and Women's Conference held in La Jolla, California, September 22-24, 1995. I, of course, spoke as a person living with the virus.

Gabby surprised me when he agreed to make a presentation to a whole room of gay women. His topic was on disclosure to family members. The women just loved his presentation and him.

Again, as in previous conferences sponsored by the group headed by Carole Norman, we were graciously treated. A San Diego newspaper also interviewed me and other women; I believe topics on disclosure are tools for educating the public but certainly at some risk. At that conference, women infected statistics were reported as: 24% as white, 54% as Black, 20% as Hispanic, 5% as Asian, and 2% as not known. As those of us in the field of HIV know, the statistics in this day and time are quite different. People of Color, including Black and Hispanic, are now at the top of the list and Whites are at the lower part of the list. And I ask: "WHAT'S WRONG WITH THIS PICTURE."

While we were in LaJolla, I became close friends with another infected woman who called herself Elizabeth. As she was married to a doctor, she did not want to use her real name. From that time, we kept in touch and saw each other at future Western Regional HIV conferences until her death in October 1998. Over the years, for me, the loss of so many women friends is the hardest part of living with this virus; I believe it's called "survivor's guilt." Instead of asking God why I was infected, my question was always, "why am I still here healthy and all; why did my friend have to die still young (in most cases). God, what do you still have in mind for me to do?" I have found the answer revealed little by little each year.

At the end of each year, as I look back of what has transpired during the year, I can see God's hand in each event I experienced; most of it is wonderful. Only deaths along the way are sad landmarks in my journey

The next three conferences Gabby and I attended in 1995 were back-to-back and all held in Los Angeles (L.A.). The first one was held October 15-18, 1995, the first Nat'l AIDS Treatment Advocates Forum sponsored by the National Association of People with AIDS (NAPWA). I learned many new tools and information to use in my new role as an AIDS advocate. Of course, many friendships were developed,

Our oldest daughter, Eunice, lived just outside of L.A. She and her then boyfriend and his parents, had a good visit while we were at the above conference.

The second conference in L.A from October 19-21, I was also sponsored to attend the National Skills Building Conference Institutes on (1) HIV Women's Issues and (2) Spirituality and HIV.

Lastly, I was invited and sponsored by NAPWA to attend the first Project Implement's American with Disability Act (ADA) training. The training was intense and taught thoroughly on the rights of the new national legislation to protect those of us infected with HIV/AIDS.

During this trip, Gabby and I also took time to go to one of our favorite TV programs, "The Price is Right. " Although we were not selected to play one of their games, we had a great time talking with folks from all over the USA who were waiting in line like us, to get tickets for one of the shows being tapped. It was like skipping school (or conference) for a day of fun. While waiting to attend the TV program, Gabby and I went next door and strolled around a huge open market; I brought home a few of the goodies I found there, especially a set to add to my salt and pepper collection.

On December 11, 1995, our youngest daughter, Anita's school paper printed a huge two-page story on HIV and featured Anita and me. It was titled, "Living with A Killer." The young man who interviewed me we had known since he and Anita attended kindergarten at a nearby Catholic school. After reading the article once it was published, I then understood more fully how positive my infection has affected my immediate family, especially our youngest, Anita, and our oldest, Roger. Although the other three children have not publically stated their views, Roger and one of his sons, Joshua, are featured in a large picture of them with Anita during an earlier AIDS walk in October, 1995. It also featured my favorite picture of Anita hugging me as I sit on our living room couch, which is draped with one of my mother's hand-crochet long shawls. To me, this is a three-generational picture of love.

The last important item of 1995 was the receipt of a video entitled, "It Could Happen to Me" which was filmed and mailed out by the AARP organization in Washington, D.C. It includes segments of my HIV presentation; however I do not know how many people have seen it nationwide; I was told it was mailed throughout the USA.

With the support from the Center for Health Policy Development (CHPD) during 1996, I attended and presented around 20 AIDS-related functions.

During March 7-9, Gabby and I attended the National Conference on Aging held in Denver, Colorado. One of the speakers was our own local Senator Gonzalo Barrientos, whom we had known since the 1960's. I served on a panel called Anciano's "Consejos" Panel (Elderly Advisory Panel). Another speaker was a man I met while I was attending U.T. at Austin. All four of us were able to have time to visit and enjoy our time off together at one time or another.

The most important memory that year happened in May 1996. Anita graduated from a local high school Academy of Science. As I recall, after her graduation, I had scheduled an interview for the both of us with a local reporter. Although I had made no firm arrangement how we would meet with the reporter, I was surprisingly impressed he found Anita and me. We answered a few of his questions, but when he asked how did Anita feel about me being able to be present with her on this special day, Anita and I both "lost" it. We both began crying almost in each other's arms. I hope I never forget that day!

Now that I've written it down, I know I won't forget it. You see, over the past several years, I have found my memory is not as it used to be. I find myself asking my husband about things/events to renew my memory; and I am not sure if this loss is due to my aging or the HIV. At any rate, I have to deal with this factor and as Gabby and I say, "Adapt, Adapt, Adapt." At times it is hard for me to do this, but I try each time it happens

The happiness did not end here. That evening our family help me plan and put together a small graduation party for Anita. The only problem was that Anita had to go to a "mandatory" dress rehearsal for the dance group that evening. If she missed the rehearsal, she would be prohibited from appearing in the final show. She was very upset her dance teacher would not make am exception. I assured Anita it would be fine; the party would still be ongoing whenever she arrived. Anita returned around 10:PM. and friends were still partying. All of a sudden, with a friend's help, Anita sat me down on a couch. and started playing a CD called "Mama," and began to perform this beautiful free style dance for me. I just sat in awe as she floated across the floor in this beautiful, green dress, tears streaming down my face! What a beautiful tribute!

This is an example of the special bond Anita and I have had all her life. I know some of her siblings can be jealous of our relationship; but what they don't realize it's because Anita and I were never sure how much time we would have together; we don't want to take it for granted. And with the other four children, I was always around for all their "firsts." Like there first day of school, their first ball game, first Browne/Girl Scout event. Graduation, marriage and best of all birth of their first baby/our grandbaby!

I must say Gabby is especially patient with me, always at my side and ready to do anything, I mean anything I ask him to do or help me do. When I'm outside gardening, he's right beside me digging a hole for my new plant, bringing me something to drink and even doing all of the cooking. I would not be in the good health I'm in were it not for him.

Before I left for Vancouver, Canada to attend the 11th International AIDS Conference July 7-12, 1996, our youngest son and his wife came to our home. What they told me was so unexpected: they came especially to say the reason they did not bring their three children (our grandchildren) over to our home more often was because they were afraid I would infect them when I kissed them. At that time, I could not believe my ears. For days I cried my heart out; Gabby could not console me.

Finally, I made a decision, which I talked over with my husband of 36 years. I told him I was going to "kill them with love." By that I meant I was going to do anything positive to see these grandchildren. We began to attend the kids' sports events; all three have been active in many sports, such as baseball, soccer, and football. I found it brings back fond memories of school events we had attended of our own five children.

When our children were young, we participated in all of their school activities; we served in all of their PTA.s often as officers. Twice, we were Presidents of their PTA's. I made baked items and sent them for special holidays. I am so proud to see this son and his wife are doing the same for their children. I've learned it is better to show love to others who have hurt you rather than hold a grudge. I often tell this son how proud I am of his parenting skills, which I know I was not good at when he was growing up, and I really mean it. I do not know if they still feel the same; it matters not. The most important thing is we continue the spirit of love my parents and in-laws showed us while they were here on earth with us.

At the end of 1996, I was proudly presented an award from Positive Threads, a local HIV newsletter at their Christmas holiday social. One of our daughters, Loretta, attended along with Gabby and me. It was such a heart-warming event in my journey with HIV.

THE CATHOLIC CHURCH AND HIV

My experience with how the Catholic Church would act and/or support or not support PWA's began in 1996. I was serving as a member of the Austin Catholic Diocese AIDS Task Force. During that year, the Task Force requested formation of a PWA focus group; the goal of this group was to meet and come up with ideas/suggestions of activities for the Task Force to undertake during the last of Task Force's three-year tenure. The PWA's did come up with some suggestions. A written report was prepared and forwarded to the Task Force. It was my understanding the report and/or its cover letter stated the PWA focus group would attend the March 1996 Task Force meeting in case questions arose to which group members could all speak to, if needed.

When I arrived at the March 1996 Task Force meeting, present were more than the usual Task Force members I had come to expect. It soon became apparent to me why they were present.

After the PWA's were seated and the meeting began, the Task Force chairperson then announced that due to a long agenda and the fact all meetings are closed to the public, the PWA focus group members present had to leave. The agenda, however, was apparently prepared the day before this meeting as it was not part of a prior mailing to me and other Task Force members. Afterwards, in a written letter after this meeting, I brought up the fact the Open Records Law requires all meetings to be open, and specifically questioned why would a Task Force meeting be closed. I also asked why so many prior non-participating Task Force members suddenly showed up for this particular meeting.

I wrote to the Task Force member (a priest) of my dismay and total shock at the lack of respect shown to me and my fellow PWA's. Also, when I looked across the table at this priest, he said nothing nor did he seem affected at all by the incident.

Tears began streaming down my face, and when my husband whispered in my ear if I wanted to leave, I responded in Spanish: "I'm not going to let this m...f...make me leave; I'm staying until the end!" It was, however, that I believed the Catholic Church had abandoned me and other PWA's as I always thought a priest to be a representative of the Church. I also wrote in my letter above, it was my experience that no action is action; thus, my conclusion of feeling abandoned by the Catholic Church. I concluded in my correspondence that future actions taken or not taken by the Church would speak for themselves on the issue outlined above. When I mailed the letter, I also sent a blind copy to the then Bishops of Austin.

Almost a year later, I received a short, curt letter by the then Bishop of the Austin Diocese, who responded to my correspondence above. I found it interesting that he questioned my understanding of Catholic theology and did not respond to the real issue I had questioned. Of course, I responded to the Bishop, however, it took me until three week later; I needed the time to vent my anger and frustration at this church leader's avoidance or misunderstanding of the real issue.

I was later able to present a training session to the Task Force; however, I believe my effort was for naught. Many of the members did not attend the meeting even though they received written notice prior to that month's meeting.

Later on in the year, my faith was restored when Gabby and I attended the 10th National Catholic HIV/AIDS Ministry Conference held in Chicago. It was our second time to attend this conference. We found it such a healing atmosphere.

THE JOURNEY CONTINUES

In 1997, I continued in my new role as what my kids called the "conference queen." A San Antonio, TX non-profit, The Center for Health Policy Development (CHPD) sponsored the first event of that year, to attend the National People of Color Living with HIV during January 23-26, held in Riverside, CA. Only Hispanic and African American PWA's attended this event. Thus began a close-knit new "family" all living with this disease. We would see each other at other conferences and future People of Color events, all in Riverside. Each time, however, we were missing those who died from the last time we were together. I know death is inevitable; however, each such loss depresses me and I go into a "blue funk" for a few days. During these times, I not only review memories I have of the person who died, but it serves as a reminder of my ultimate fate. It's not the fear of death, but more of the anticipated horror of how I will die.

For over a decade, San Francisco was the scene of the annual HIV National AIDS Update Conference. Gabby and I first attended this conference from March 18-22, 1997. We were sponsored by San Antonio's CHPD AIDS organization. Going to San Francisco was like a vacation for us. Each year we attended the conference, we stayed in the same hotel, had breakfast across the street at the same little restaurant owned by an oriental family, who were always gracious and kind. Of course our favorite thing to do was to ride the trolley to and from Pier 39. We loved our time together in San Francisco during each March, which afforded many opportunities to purchase additions to my salt/pepper collection at home.

At the end of the above conference, I conducted an AIDS workshop on HIV and Aging at the 2nd National Association of HIV over Fifty (NAHOF) one-day conferences.

Throughout the remainder of 1997, I partici-pated in another 20+ HIV-related activities and conferences.

Some of these are discussed below.

On April 18, 1997, I appeared in an NMAC report on Parity, Inclusion and Representation (PIR), which discusses the need for infected people of all races and gender need "to be at the table." This means all of us need to be part of decision-making processes on services and programs for those of us infected with the virus.

At the request of Sally Weiss, I wrote an article for the ADA Crosswalk magazine, regarding how the American with Disabilities ACT can help persons living with HIV/AIDS.

On June 2,1997, I was asked to be a speaker at the National Association of People with AIDS in Reno, Nevada; however, there was no spare time for gambling!

I also appeared in a national magazine, POZ, in an article entitled, "Profile Mother Mary," which was published in July 1997.

Our next conference July 17-22, 1997, was held in Chicago again at the National Catholic AIDS Conference (NCAN) entitled, Companions on the Journey. We have a great group picture of the 1997 Planning Team Gabby and I were asked to serve on. Our efforts in planning this conference were well received; all the planning committee received many praises by many of the attendees. We continued to attend this conference each year in July thereafter until 2004. Afterwards, Gabby and I were so touched to receive a personal letter each from Vice President Al Gore's wife's Advisor on HIV, Miguel Bustos, to thank us for our efforts on the NCAN conference, which he also attended.

One of my fondest memories of this particular conference is when a young woman named, Martha Hesskew, arrived at the conference for the first time. She was in tears and asking everyone to find "Mary Moreno." Martha, who was in her 30's, was one of the women in our HIV women's group in Austin, Women Raising. When I came upon Martha, she fell into my arms crying and complaining about the horrible taxi driver who was angry because his fare was $26 and Martha only had $25; he threatened to call the police, but then changed his mind and threw her luggage on the steps and left. That was the last time Martha would have to worry about money while at this conference and all future NCAN conferences. She made friends so easily and never left without a few extra dollars. She never asked for help; we all just loved her and wanted to make her journey a little better.

Martha attended as many of the conference workshops as she could, but her favorite part was the banquet and dance held the last night of the event. She laughingly made fun of our yearly "chicken" or whatever dinner we were served, and she could hardly wait for the dance to begin. It was held in another building; Martha was always the first one on the dance floor. And did I tell you, Martha was usually the last one to go back to her room.

The first time Gabby and I attended the banquet and dance, we realized how different and yet similar to dances we had attended in the past. Everyone was having fun dancing; and it was the first time we experienced men dancing with men as well as women dancing with women.

It all seemed so "natural" there in Chicago at Loyola University on Lake Michigan, but as I said, it was Gabby and my first time to be a part of such a joyful occasion.

For several years thereafter, one of the waiters at the banquet would stay after dinner to dance with Martha. She loved to dance---any dance and every dance. Always the life of the party! In actuality, I believe it was the only time Martha really had fun that whole year. Martha's marriage was not a happy one; her husband was very verbally abusive. Even our doctor (who was also Martha's doctor and specializes in HIV) would lecture Martha's husband on her needs, often to no avail.

You see Martha was from a rural little town near San Antonio, very poor and infected with AIDS. Diagnosed when her youngest daughter was born around 1992, Martha's story was like so many new infections: young women between the ages of 24-35. Martha soon became like a daughter to Gabby and me. She called us Mom and Dad and with her doctor's knowledge, often stayed at our home upon released from many hospitalizations. Martha's doctor is also Gabby and my doctor, and he would often tell her: "Go home with Mary and Gabby and have an ice cream snack and watch TV." She had already lost her baby daughter to AIDS on December 25, 1995. Maratha, however, did have an older daughter, Jessica, from an earlier partner. Martha's wish was to stay healthy at least until her daughter Jessica's graduation from high school. But for whatever reason(s), it was not in God's plan. Martha died on May 16,2004. a year before Jessica's graduation. And Jessica never finished high school.

It was not the first time I endured the loss of a women friend to AIDS; each time it's like I loose a part of me. I have counted about 12 women who have died since I co-founded Women Rising. After each death, I wonder how many more souls would be lost to this horrendous disease before it's all over with.

I spoke about this loss in a speech I gave during the previous year's (1997) NCAN Conference. It is worth repeating here:

"I am one of the new faces of HIV/AIDS: a woman …and a woman of color . . .My spiritual journey with this new Life Partner began in February 1984, two weeks after I was infected with HIV from a blood transfusion I received during a hysterectomy, when for the first tune I picked up our family Bible and began reading the Book of Job. I did not understanding the meaning of God's new presence in my life until I experienced so much hate and fear from my fellow co-workers when they became aware of my infection. During one of these dark moments, I even asked 'God, why have you forsaken me.' Then I followed with' 'If you do help me Lord Jesus, Do it quickly.

"I soon began to see and understand God working through me and when I won the first HIV court case in my community, I felt so blessed and thankful. And I soon learned, God was Not finished with me. He then offered opportunities for me to move from a preoccupation with law and justice to a disposition of love. This over-whelming love help heal the wounds from losing my job, rejuvenate my self-confidence and pride lost during those struggles, and led me to new and more fulfilling work in HIV. For the past two, almost three years, my focus has been on HIV women's issues and spirituality. Successes gained on women's issues fostered false confidence. Stumbling blocks on planned spirituality activities aroused old feelings of doubt, mistrust. Again I questioned God's presence. I just could not understand why my plan was not succeeding. Don't people with this virus deserve God in their lives? Why do so-called Christians show so much fear and hate towards us? With God's help I am sure the answers will come . . .quickly Lord before we all die in Vain!"

The following year, from April 30 to May 3, 1998, the National Association of People with AIDS (NAPWA) held its National Survival Training, "Staying Alive" just outside of Washington, D.C., at a Hilton Hotel in Crystal City, VA. Quite unexpected to me, I arrived at our first meeting with a terrible itch on my waist. As I was in a small group of women only, they asked me to pick up my shirt. When I did, several of them shouted out together: "SH N G L E S, you've got shingles." As they were explaining what it was, several of the women began pulling out medicines they had in their purses and offering them to me. Upon returning home and a visit with my HIV doctor, he told me how lucky I was to have received medications so soon after coming down with the disease. I was well shortly thereafter.

Shingles occurs only to persons who as a child had chicken pox. And now I recall when some of my kids had an outbreak of chicken pox, how I hoped all of them would get the disease to "get it over with it." What a joke on me!

Even after this experience, I didn't realize how painful this disease could be until I was reinfected last year (2005). I learned Shingles affects one's nervous system. I ended up going to a pain management specialist for shots in my back to deaden the nerves to my right side/limbs (arm, leg hand and foot).

To this day, August 24,2006, I am still under a doctor's care for the remaining pain from the last bout with shingles. I also am being treated for neuropathy in my right hand, which after various treatments is now being diagnosed as corporal tunnel and will require surgery. My hope is I finish this book before that event in order to give a copy as a gift to each of our children this Christmas.

Now, back to events of 1998. The next big conference I attended May 12-15,1998 was here in Austin, TX. Again, on full scholarship, I attended the 11th Texas HIV/STD Conference held at the Hyatt Regency Hotel. . Many of my friends from Austin as well as San Antonio were there and we had a blast talking and hanging out together. We especially enjoyed the talent show put on by many of the conference participants at a local restaurant. Friends included Mary Helen Gloria and "Tiny Yoli" Yolanda, who founded and serves as the coordinator of her HIV women's group, Mujeres Unidas. For some, it was their first major conference to attend.

Many women of our local Women Rising group were there, and as I watched them during workshops, it was apparent they were learning a lot. They asked questions and listened intently.

That summer, Gabby and I each received a scholarship to our beloved NCAN Conference entitled: WHO IS MY NEIGHBOR, held July 16-21, in Chicago at Loyola University in Chicago. Our oldest daughter, Eunice also was a scholarship recipient and shared a room with Monica. Johnson. Those two hit it off right away; they were always together, going and coming. They remained friends to this day.

That year at the NCAN conference I was a presenter of a workshop, "The Changing Faces of AIDS: People Over Age 50." I included handouts and a short synopsis of my experience living with HIV and showed a film compiled by AARP called "It Could Happen to Me" I believe it was too personal for Eunice as she left the room during the presentation. Later, she told me how sad it made her feel.

It was quiet shocking for our daughter to meet another "Eunice." as our daughter always believed she would never find another person with the same name. Actually, she met Eunice Tate, from District Heights, MD. While Ms. Tate is 4 ft 11 inches and often wears a blonde wig, our Eunice is 5 ft.9 inches and slim with dark hair and quite different;

Our Eunice and Monica especially enjoyed the evening hospitality time. Each night we had different snacks and a raffle. All day long, we would hear assigned participants call out, "Tickets! Tickets!" Our favorite raffle seller was Father Nick Christiana or "Nick" as we all called him .He was so full of life and laughter. Later in 2001, we learned he died from a heart attack and we were all divested. We held a memorial for Nick at the following year's NCAN conference.

A month after returning from Chicago, I received notice of another scholarship to attend the National Association of People with AIDS (NAPWA)'s "Helping Communities Build Leadership Regional Training." in New Orleans from August 28-30, 1998. Getting together with old friends was fantastic; the training, as usual, was excellent. The only problem for me was finding a restaurant, which served non-spicy food. With all the medications I had taken over the past 10 years or so, my stomach could only cope with just salt and pepper. Period! Otherwise, I would be in the bathroom a lot, and I mean a LOT! Except for this, I loved going to New Orleans and have been there many, many times.

On September 16, 1998, I was featured in the Commentary" section of the Austin American-Statesman (Pg. A14 &15), entitled, "One of the 'new faces' of AIDS, written by Susan Richardson. The article was written to advertise a two-day conference listed below. It spoke about my experiences living with the virus.

In September (17 & 18), 1998, I was invited to be a speaker at the first WOMEN OF COLOR HIV/AIDS PREVENTION & TREATMENT Conference here in Austin, TX. Sponsored by the Center for Health Training. My session was entitled, "Surfacing confidence and satisfaction within ourselves." Although I was already aware of the need to focus on this issue, this was the first time it was being addressed if only at the local arena. Again, many of my friends from San Antonio's Mujeres Unidas were there, some like me, served as presenters.

From October 10-12, 1998, the National Minority AIDS Council (NMAC) provided a scholarship for me to attend their Southwestern Regional Advocacy Training for Women of Color in Albuquerque, NM. Sharing ideas and experiences with other women of color like my friends from San Antonio, Mary Helen, Tiny Yoli, and others was like more of a "girls night out" We took in all the training information, but we also took time for fun and hanging out together. Oh yes, we found time to do some shopping. We even had a dress up Halloween party. All had a great time!

When I was asked to serve on an ongoing national HIV work group almost two years earlier, I really thought I could make a difference. The group was reviewing problems identified at the 1994 national HIV conference; and the end product would be recommendations to present to the directors of many federal agencies.. I was asked to join the group around 1996.

Our final report was scheduled to be presented at the Second US Conference on AIDS held at the Adams Mark Hotel in Dallas from October 29 trough November 1,1998. In addition, I was invited to participate in a 1-day Latino Critical Issues Institute October 29th. My participation in part of this process was exuberating and I must say, self-satisfying. I was so looking forward to our planned presentation. But, it was not to be!

On the morning of the NMAC proposed presentation of the National Minority HIV Plan, all members of our workgroup were called together and we were told our presentation had been called off by "the powers to be." In its place would be the announcement of the First African American AIDS Initiative in the USA. You could hear a hush come over us. Then, thank goodness, the selected leaders of each subgroup began talking, saying we were not going to fight amongst ourselves. We anticipated that was what was expected from us. Instead, we began talking how best to handle this catastrophe.

At this point, I "LOST" IT. I became so angry; I just rushed out of that room and ran until as usual, I could find Gabby! Tears were rolling down my face. Friends I met along the way tried to stop and comfort me.. I could only think of my fellow PWAs who died throughout this process, some who were here that day were probably on their last days here on this earth. AND FOR WHAT?!

Quite naturally, the rest of the conference had no meaning to me. Gabby just tried to make my stay there as comfortable as possible.

When I received a Certificate of Appreciation from the federal Office of Minority Health for my participation in the work group, sighed October 30, 1998, my first instinct was to throw it into our recycle box; but later I took it out of the box and filed it in one of my binders.

While I was attending this conference, I was given a note; someone from San Pedro, CA. was trying to reach me. It turned out to be from my friend, Elizabeth's husband. He was calling to let Gabby and me know of Elizabeth's death. Elizabeth had specially asked him to call me. I only felt sadness at loosing another friend to AIDS. Just this past month, I lost another woman friend, Kim. She was my roommate, at each of the WOMEN RISING 3-day retreats I attended. I will miss her laughter and warmth.

Two months later, I was a speaker at the WORLD AIDS DAY ceremony at the request of Austin's Interfaith Care Alliance. I spoke on "What Community Means to Me," The thank-you letter I received from the Director of the Care Alliance, David Smith, a few days afterwards help my spirit soar once again. He is such a kind and wonderful person; I would do anything for him…well almost anything!

I also received two other certificates; (1) from the then Mayor of Austin, Kirk Watson, for my service on the Austin Area Comprehensive HIV Planning Council, and (2) another one from the Mayor, A Community Service award, also for my participation on the HIV Planning Council.

Then on December 8, 1998, I wrote a letter to the Chair of the HIV Planning Council. I outlined my concerned for the lack of commitment by the Council to allocate dollars to what I believed was the real need: people of color, in particular women of color. Instead, the Council voted not to allocate $563,000 to support outreach services for African American women with a drug addiction background, but instead to allocate $75,000 to fund procurement of consultant services to conduct a study/analysis of the HIV delivery system. (Whatever that means.) I know this may not be understandable or of concern to the everyday citizen, but to those of us living with this virus as a new lifelong partner, it can mean the future of our fellow neighbors.

Towards the end of that year, I received an extra nice Christmas gift. On December 25, 1998, *The Austin American Statesman* wrote an article entitled, "Mary Moreno, Facing HIV and AIDS head on," with a picture of my granddaughter, Rachel Lyles, and me. I then received a letter of recognition from our district House of Representative member, Llyod. Doggett. For me, it was a wonderful way to end the year in spite of all the struggles I endured that year.

The next year began with me again going to San Francisco to attend the 11th National HIV/AIDS Update Conference. It was held March 23-26, 1999, and the Center for Health Policy Development (CHPD) of San Antonio, TX. sponsored and paid for all expenses related to this trip. Not only did this trip afford me the opportunity to learn new HIV/AIDS strategies in my role as educator regarding all aspects of the disease, I also had the opportunity to be with conference friends from all over the USA.

From April 6-9, 1999, I was awarded a scholarship to attend the 12th Annual TEXAS HIV/STD Conference held here in Austin. It was held at our new Austin Convention Center. This conference provided me the opportunity to speak on the creation of the first Central Texas HIV Women's Group, ***WOMEN RISING*** which provides a safe place to discuss issues, participate in art, and other therapy projects or just sit and visit. Attendees were asking a lot of questions and showed interest in forming a similar program in their communities. It warmed my heart to witness so much interest in our organization.

On April 27, 1999, Gabby drove us to San Antonio, TX. I was invited to participate on an HIV panel to discuss issues facing Hispanics regarding living with and staying healthy with the HIV/AIDS virus.

The next major event was held May 26-29, 1999, in Tempe, Arizona. I served as a speaker at one of the plenary entitled "People LIVING with AIDS - A Multigenerational Prospective." I also spoke as a Board member of a San Antonio's HIV women's group in a workshop entitled "Latina PWA Empowerment." The focus was on "how-to" build capacity skills. I found this conference to be one of the best I've attended and it followed true to form to the theme entitled: "El Tapiz: Weaving a Healthy Latino Community." It was great to meet new Latinas/os with similar interests as mine. Plus, we found time to meet and learn each other's stories.

During July 22-27, 1999, Gabby and I attended the 12th annual NCAN HIV/AIDS Ministry Conference entitled "Prophetic Voices," again on scholarships. I always look forward to this particular conference; it provided peace and rest as well as time with old friends and opportunities to make new ones. I conducted a workshop focused on the spiritual needs of women over age 50 living with H/AIDS and described components of a successful strategy that one could implement as a new program, reinvigorate or renew an ongoing one. Pictures of this event reflect the joy and wonderful spirit of this conference; more importantly, the peace Gabby and I experienced once again!

There were three more conferences I attended in 1999. The South Texas AIDS Training (STAT) Project invited me to present a workshop, "Latinas Living with AIDS" at the September 10, 1999 at the 7th Annual HIV/AIDS Update Conference in South Padre Island. In addition to the workshops that were invigorating, we also took time for fun in the facility's swimming pool with friends from the San Antonio HIV group, "Mujeres Unida Contra El Sida."

From September 1999, to September 2001. I served as a member of the Texas State Community planning Group (CPG). The purpose of the group was to identify gaps in needs of PWAs (People living with AIDS/HIV) and make recommendations for future programs to ensure these gaps are closed. With almost 60 members from all parts of Texas, with very strong opinions, we had to work hard to reach consensus on many arenas. I found it a great opportunity to gain new skills and friendships.

The Center for Health Policy Development (CHPD) of San Antonio then invited me to attend the National Latino AIDS Voice (NLAV) Legislative Briefing to the Congressional Hispanic Caucus members as well as a press conference held September 29, 1999 in Washington, D.C. NLAV was composed of Latino AIDS service providers from around the country to advocate on critical issues involving the Latino community and HIV/AIDS.

I served on a PWA panel to speak as a Latina living with HIV and barriers I had encountered. In addition, staff of CHPD took me along to make visits to selected Hispanic congressional offices in D.C. to provide a new prospective on HIV/AIDS in the Latino community and to offer concrete legislative proposals to address this crisis.

During October 9-12, 1999, I again received a scholarship to attend the first National Conference on Women and HIV/AIDS, held in Los Angeles, CA. I found it quiet an experience! The theme of the conference was entitled, "Navigating into the new millennium through collaboration." I also served as a committee member for the National Community Advisory Board for the conference.

Expecting 4,000 or so attendees, it became very chaotic as almost daily, more and more women arrived to the conference. We learned later that as the conference sponsors received donations, women who had not been invited prior to the start of the conference, were being contacted and arrangements made to fly them to the conference. It appeared, however, that no pre-planned adjustments were anticipated nor made for the increased numbers. This resulted in shortages of food advertised for participants, and "all hell broke loose," particularly in (sad to say) the African American attendees. They were rude, obnoxious and jut out mean! In the end, many of us were unable to be fed and we had to go outside of the conference site and purchase a meal.

I was a presenter on October 10th along with the Director of CHPD. Just prior to the presentation, I had a misunderstanding with our oldest daughter who lives in L.A. and became so upset, I had difficulty composing myself prior to the presentation. My roommate, Martha, was a Godsend; she did everything she could to calm me down. In addition to this incident, I ended up loosing my purse while Martha and I were eating in a nearby diner. That was really divesting until Charlene of CHPD loaned me some money to make it through the conference. That was one conference I wished Gabby were with me; he would have kept me on track with my money. Although the subjects covered during the conference were interesting and excellent, all the struggles I underwent overshadowed the enjoyment of the conference. I was so glad when I returned to Austin, and back at home with Gabby.

In November 1999, I attended our local Women Rising yearly retreat. It was such an opportunity to relax and be with old friends; the retreat itself was so healing for me.

On December 1, 1999, I participated at the yearly AIDS Day activities, along with Martha and her family. I also met up with one of my cousins I had not seen in over 20 years; we took time to visit and "catch up."

In the December 1999 issue of the WORLD NEWSLETTER, Anita and I were featured in an article I wrote for Rebecca Dennison, "Why Not Me God?" A short article about my life living with the disease, I especially enjoy reading the last part of the article: "This year, Moreno's youngest child, Anita turned 22 years and brought her first home (in San Antonio). When the family went out to dinner to celebrate, Anita said, 'Well Mom…We made another milestone."

That same month, I received the final revision of the "Texas HIV Reporting by Name." I had served as a member of the Community Consultation Group. The group was formed in the summer of 1998, and met throughout 1998 to discuss issues associated with community reactions to the proposed HIV reporting system. I was asked to serve as a person living with HIV/AIDS. The majority of the members of this group did not agree with HIV reporting by name; however, we did agree to work and discuss matters assuming that the Texas Board of Health would approve rule changes to allow HIV reporting by name. The meetings and discussions of the group were not devoted to whether HIV reporting was desirable, but focused on what the rule change would mean for their communities, and how to prepare their communities and clients for the change. As it turned out, HIV reporting was implemented smoothly in Texas, without disruption of local prevention efforts. Those of us infected with the virus believed our efforts working on this work group were well worth the effort.

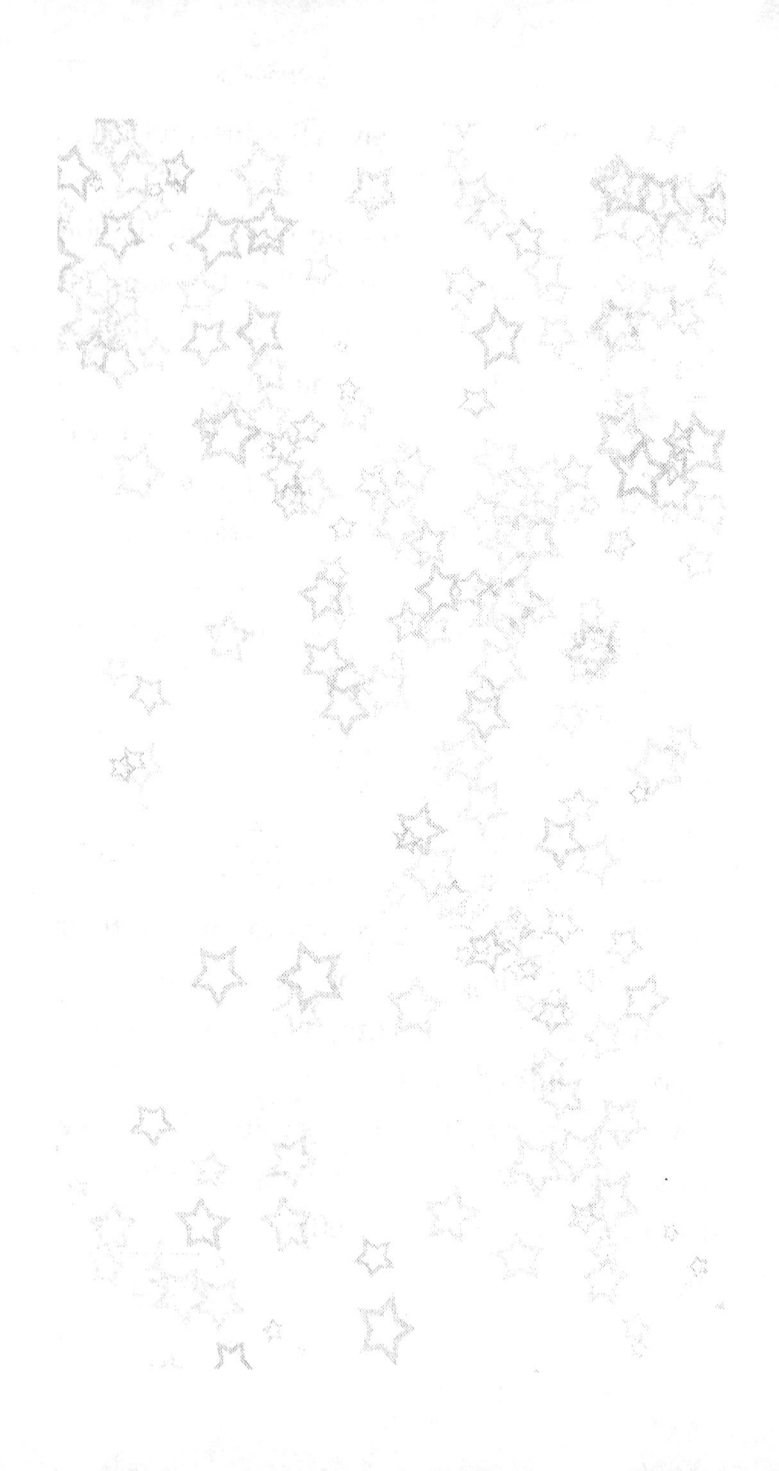

INTO THE NEW MILLENNIUM

The year 2000 begins a new era and time to reflect on the last part of my life with a new lifelong companion called HIV. I find myself amazed that after 16 years, I am still alive and doing okay health wise. I do miss my many friends who have died; sometimes I feel very lonely, and I feel guilty for feeling this way. During these times, I just sit (usually outside on my back porch) and say a few prayers for all of my friends who have passed and I ask God to give me the strength to keep going forward. I also thank God for the unfailing love of my husband, Gabby. He has been my rock; even though it took us a long time to get to the place we are now, I believe it was all worth the effort. Many people may not know or understand our love for each other; I only know God knew when He brought Gabby and me together that Spring of 1959. And to think we only dated a few months before we realized how much we loved each other. We got engaged on Friday, November 13, 1959, and married the following Valentine's Day, February 14,1960 at a Catholic church in San Antonio, TX.

The first event of 2000 included my participation on an HIV panel at the "HIV/AIDS in the New Millennium Conference. It was held in Laredo, Texas on January 28, 2000. I was one of three panelists who spoke on our experience on the topic "HIV, Women and Families. The question and answer session afterwards involved a lot of discussion with the audience. I found the people in the Valley very warm and friendly not standoffish as others north of Texas

The next event was a leadership Training Institute "Issues Facing Women with HIV/AIDS." It was held on March 7, 2000 at the CHPD office in San Antonio, TX. A representative from the DUPONT Pharmaceutical Company spoke on how to keep ourselves healthy and abreast of upcoming HIV Issues

The next conference both Gabby and I attended was our annual trip to San Francisco, to attend the 12th annual National HIV/AIDS Conference held by AMFAR AIDS Research from March 14-17. 2000. As usual the information presented was so valuable and easy to understand. And of course, Gabby and I did our usual trip on the famous trolley to and from Pier 39 to purchase more goodies for our youngest child and an addition to my salt & pepper collection.

The next event was a second Leadership Training Institute on "Issues Facing Women with HIV/AIDS" held in San Antonio, TX from June 20-22, 2000. Again, it was sponsored by the DUPONT Pharmaceuticals Company in collaboration also with the Department of Health and Human Services, the Office of Minority Health-Resource Center, the Office of Women's Health, Region VI, and San Antonio's Center for Health Policy Development (CHPD). I served on the planning committee as well as a Panelist on the "Barriers to Treatment." My panel's focus was how to overcome barriers and become adherent to treatment to benefit those of us living with HIV/AIDS. I found this topic of extreme interest to me. After so many years of taking HIV medications (meds), it has become difficult for me to adhere to the daily regiment; often, it's so easy just to not take the dozen or so pills each night.

The next conference was held in Arlington, Virginia, just outside of D.C., from June 26-27, 2000. It was called "Empowerment Summit, Eliminating Disparities in HIV/AIDS, Health Outcomes Among Women of Color" sponsored by the National Minority AIDS Council (NMAC). It was described as a working conference and attendance was by Invitation-only. I felt very blessed when I received a letter of invitation from the NMAC (National Minority AIDS Council) of Washington, D.C. to attend this conference with expenses paid by NMAC.

The focus of this conference was very unique. The women were placed in small groups; each group reviewed a list of questions related to women issues. During the discussions in my group, I found it astonishing and at the same time, so blessed and comforting that in my community in Austin, TX, we have so many services that are not available in other parts of the USA. In addition to client services at most of the organizations, the largest AIDS agency in town (ASA) also supports a dental clinic just for infected clients, and they do all types of dental care services and the cost is based on individual incomes. Over the past 10 years, specific services for women and men have been available at ASA. One of the women's projects was the formation of the first Central Texas women's group another woman and I co-founded called Women Raising. It was formed in the spring of 1994, with the guidance of Rebecca Dennison from Oakland, CA.. Rebecca and I met back in 1990 at the first Western Region HIV Women's Conference, held in La Jolla, CA. I saw Rebecca again while attending the International Conference on AIDS in Yokahama, Japan. It was while in Japan, that I approached Rebecca about wanting to start a women's program similar to hers in CA. She graciously agreed to help with our first retreat, and took part in the retreat, which was held in April 1995.

I felt so blessed to see the fruitarian of a goal I had for a long time, and I am grateful to both my co-founder, Sylvia Lopez and Rebecca Dennison. Since that first retreat, retreats are now held every year in November. If funds are available, we may have several one-day retreats throughout the year. These retreats usually include an art project, lunch, and other activities such as dance lessons, Massage, acupuncture, journaling how-to and mask making. We have a fantastic group of women volunteers who serve as staff. These women work at HIV and other social agencies throughout Travis County (mostly Austin) and each has their own special talents. They are the backbone of Women Rising. Without them, our women's group would not be in existence this day.

Another positive of attending this conference was, as in past conferences, being with friends in the HIV arena. One of my favorite people is an HIV/AIDS social worker from New York, Suki Ports. Suki and I have worked on HIV/AIDS issues for more years than I can remember. I admire her tenacity and friendship Pictures I have on file of this conference reflect all the beautiful women whom I now know and respect.

The 13th annual National Catholic AIDS Network (NCAN) conference's theme was called, "Proclaim Jubilee" As usual, it was held at Loyola University Chicago, Ill., from July 20-25, 2000. I was asked to present a workshop, which I called

"The Changing Faces of AIDS: People over Age 50." I spoke about how the virus is impacting the older generation, how symptoms are misdiagnosed with symptoms of aging by health providers, why people in this age group do not believe it is important to be tested for this disease. I also identified strategies to include in informational booklets in programs throughout all states At the end of the workshop, I showed AARP's video "It Could Happen to Me," which shared interviews of individuals in this age group and how they were infected. I was pleased the workshop received a high evaluation score by the attendees

The pictures I took show the faces of many of our friends; one is of our Eunice with the conference "Eunice" and the fun we had in the hospitality room during each night's prize drawings. Others we shared fun with included Mary of Comfort House in the Valley, Sister Rose, of South Bend, Ind. Michelle Bennington, who runs an HIV ministry program in Charlotte, N.C., Ana Mendoza of San Antonio; Sister Mary Annel from El Salvador (who brought beautiful and memorable hand-made Crosses made by her AIDS group from her country to sell to conferees;

Miguel Bustos from San Francisco, CA, and our own "Martha" Hesskew (our "extra" daughter) The fact is there are too many people who attend this yearly conference to list here. All of them come up to us throughout the time we spend together, with a big hug and a kiss on the cheek.

Mary Rincones, The Director of Comfort House in McAllen, TX invited Gabby and me to conduct a workshop on October 21, 2000. Gabby and I were well received by the participants as we spoke on our experiences as an infected wife and as a caregiver. Afterwards, we had a wonderful lunch and time to visit with the audience on an individual basis. It was a great experience for both Gabby and me.

The last activity of 2000, was an article written about me in the National HIV Over Fifty organization's newsletter, NAHOF CONNECTION, "ONE WOMAN'S JOURNEY." It featured a 4-column report of my journey with HIV. In addition, I was asked as in other conferences, what available prevention programs were there for seniors? My thought was: What prevention programs? In anticipation of this question, I did identify some strategies/suggestions I came up with that can be included in future AIDS awareness activities for this age group.

Again, as in past years, Gabby and I traveled to San Francisco, CA., March 20-23, 2001, to attend AMFAR's 13th National HIV/AIDS Update Conference. In addition to attending workshops, I was invited to conduct a workshop, "HIV and later Life: Creating Caring Partnerships" along with other members of the National Association on HIV Over Fifty (NAHOF). I focused on how my life with HIV included an awakening of the spiritual side of my life and the positive effects that have resulted.

On this trip, our youngest daughter, Anita, and her boyfriend, Robert Gutierrez, accompanied us. It made me so happy to have them with us. You see, they were just beginning to date again after breaking up more than a year earlier. During the time they were not together, Robert had moved to Kansas City and was still working at a major airline, would fly to Austin to visit Gabby and me. Robert and I had long talks; he admitted he was mainly responsible for the breakup, and asked for my advice what he could do to get Anita back. Both Gabby and I had long agreed it best not to interfere in our children's lives, unless asked. I don't remember exactly what I told Robert, but in general I told him he had to gain Anita's trust again. Robert must have taken my advice to heart, because they eventually were a couple again, and were married in Las Vegas, Thursday, January 9, 2003, with family and close friends, followed by a good ole' Mexican Wedding Reception and Dance two days later (Jan. 11th) at their Catholic Church in San Antonio.

Meanwhile, back to San Francisco, after the conference concluded, we spent an extra day or two to visit Napa Valley, the wine country, as well as the Red Woods. It was an awesome excursion. Although Anita later told me at times she was uneasy, I couldn't tell. At the time, I just believed these two were meant to be together, and look at them now: married and with a beautiful daughter, 1 of our 8 grandchildren.

Returning home from the conference in San Francisco, I made plans to attend the 13th Texas HIV/STD Conference here in Austin, April 16-20, 2001 Although I was not a presenter, I attended several workshops on interrupting taking medications. This was of great interest to me because after so many years of taking different HIV meds, it was becoming more and more difficult to be adherent to my schedule. I believe I have been blessed to still be as healthy as I am dealing with this problem all the time. Even now, September 19, 2006, I still struggle to take my daily meds. Thank God I have Gabby to prod me every night to "don't forget to take your pills," or "have you taken your pills tonight?" Sometimes I feel like saying, "Stop! Stop!" But as I know it's out of love for me, I just ask Gabby to bring me a glass of juice and I drown my 15 or so pills.

Our next conference was not until June 22-23, 2001, in Boston, Maryland, to attend the 4th National Conference n HIV/AIDS and Aging. We were sponsored by NAHOF and I served as co-chair of the conference with Jim Campbell. I also spoke as a panelist on "HIV Women Over 50 Years and spirituality," provided suggestions to incorporate in current education programs by ASO's (AIDS Service Organizations) and included my personal story.

On June 30, 2001, I was one of the first graduating Class of our HIV women's group, Women Rising's Rising Star University. We even had a graduation ceremony at our local Hyatt Regency Hotel, diplomas and all. You can see our proud and smiling faces in a group picture we had taken of us. My closest friends, Betty, Martha, Donna, Melissa, and the other co-founder, Sylvia Lopez, all were part of this very memorable day; I shall carry them in my heart forever.

On our next trip, Gabby and I both received scholarships to attend the 14th NCAN Conference, July 19-24, 2001 at Loyola University on Lake Michigan in Chicago. I received a cute note from the registrar, Frederick, "Remember to take the plane to Chicago."

Frederick's note reminded me of the phopah I did the year before. I was very involved with so many activities, when I made plane reservations for our summer conference; I mistakenly booked us a flight to New York instead of to Chicago. It wasn't until Gabby and I were about to get off the airplane, we realized we were in New York. Not to worry, I thought. I'll just go up to the ticket counter and tell the agent what I did and get us a ticket to Chicago. NOT!!! I soon realized how difficult was my request and how costly. I finally resulted to my standby plea, "I've been

HIV+ from a blood transfusion I received 13 years ago, bla, bla, bla!" Well, it worked, the agent saw how desperate we were and after talking to her supervisor, she said she could give us both a ticket to Chicago for a total of $500. (That was better than the original quote of $1,000+). I instantly gave her my American Express card and we were on our way back to Chicago, and I said prayers of thanksgiving all the way. From then on Gabby is now in charge of reviewing our airline tickets to ensure we are on the correct flight. And, of course, he enjoyed telling the story to everyone at the NCAN Conference that year.

Once we were settled in at the Conference, we found relaxation, comfort and peace of mind with our friends there, including Betty Mitchell from Austin, Martha Hesskew from Blanco, Mary Rincones from McAllen, Michelle Bennington from North Carolina, Fr. Nick (our TICKETS seller) and many more. Gabby and I took Martha on the "L" (subway) to Chinatown where Martha bought a few knickknacks for her family, and Betty joined us. Of course, the end of the dinner and dance was as much fun as in past years; Martha danced her feet off and had a blast.

Then Came September 11, 2001, and ...

LIFE AS IT WAS BEFORE, WAS NO LONGER

Gabby and I decided to cancel our scheduled flight to Los Angeles to attend and present at the 7th Annual Latino Behavioral Health Institute. We based our decision not only on the terrorists' attack on the Twin Towers in New York, but also the fear there could be more attacks on the wet coast.

We did, however, drive to San Antonio, TX. to attend NMAC's Regional Training, October 2-5, 2001 at the St. Anthony Hotel. Again, Gabby and I interacted and ate with friends from Mujeres Unidas. Of course, we talked about the events of 9/11/2001, and how it affected each of us.

Although I received a scholarship to the AMFAR's 14th National HIV/AIDS Update Conference in San Francisco, March 19-22, 2002,

I became too ill to take the trip. I was a little disappointed, but I believe it more important to address health issues first and foremost.

While I did not attend the Texas HIV Connection 8th Annual 2002 Street Outreach Worker's Conference held June 16-19, 2002, I did loan two homemade little spirit dolls I made during our Women Rising 3-day retreats. The staff asked for these dolls to reflect samples of some of the art projects performed at these retreats.

On our next trip, we flew to Loyola University on Lake Michigan, in Chicago, to attend the 15th NCAN HIV/AIDS Ministry Conference held July 18-23, 2002. We were embraced by many friends including Michelle Bennington of N. Carolina, our beloved leaders, Frederick (registrar), Fr. Rodney and many more to AIDS.

Our next trip was September 19-22, 2002. We received a scholarship to attend U.S. CONFERENCE ON AIDS held in Anaheim, CA. Unlike previous conferences, this one included "Institutes" on specific topics. I attended the Institute on Women and HIV/AIDS: The Face of women and HIV/AIDS. I attended this institute and found it very interesting; however, it was geared more towards persons who needed skills to begin their work as an advocate.

While Gabby and I were at the conference, he became ill. I took him to the conference's PWA Infirmary. The nurse on duty took Gabby's blood pressure and a diabetes blood test. She then advised I should take Gabby to an ER ASAP. We then contacted our oldest daughter, Eunice, who lives 20 minutes away; she drove us to the nearest Medical center. The staff there was fantastic; we received excellent care, picked up some prescriptions for Gabby and went home to Eunice's apartment. As we had pre-planned to stay an extra day to visit with Eunice, it gave us time for Gabby's meds to start working. Our concern was to help Gabby get his blood pressure down to the point there would be no danger for him while flying.

After arriving home, we made a doctor's appointment for the next day for an exam.

Yea! Good news. Tests showed Gabby was doing okay; we were given newer prescriptions and scheduled a follow-up visit in two weeks. Now, four years later, Gabby is doing so well, he is now the stronger of the two of us. I'm praying and hoping that after my corporal tunnel surgery on my right hand, I will be "good to go."

This incident reminds me why I appreciate and value so much the medical care Gabby and I receive. But this is not the case in all states, and that makes me so sad for the folks living in these states with this horrendous virus.

At the request of the National Episcopal AIDS Coalition, I spoke at their Conference held October 11-12, 2002, at the Radisson Hotel. I gave a 30-minute talk on my experiences living as a Latina with HIV, and the struggles I overcame. I received a $200 donation to the Women Rising project. It was a very unexpected donation, which was put towards expenses left from the past month's 3-day retreat.

The last event I participated in that year, I spoke at the State Capitol HIV/AIDS Rally held October 19,2002. Senator Gonzalo Barrientos of Austin sponsored it. Senator Barrientos has always been a strong supporter of the AIDS epidemic. The purpose of the rally was a public awareness message of the urgent need for funding for HIV/AIDS programs, especially targeted to women of color: Latinas and African-Americans. In addition.

one of the speakers told of the rising numbers especially in the African-American females with a drug addiction and/or living with someone doing drugs and the risks involved.

As I said before, after 9/11/01, my days as an active HIV/AIDS Educator went to a screeching slow down, but not totally out. The few conferences we attended included the following

Gabby and I spent July 15,2003 at the National Council of La Raza, at the Hyatt Hotel in Austin, TX. I spoke as a Latina presenter infected with HIV, to tell the health issues I have experienced.

That year, Gabby and I were able to make our annual Chicago trip to attend the 16th National Catholic HIV/AIDS Ministry Conference held July 17-22, 2003. As usual, it was a very restful and healing time.I was so touched when Martha asked me to help place an AIDS quilt panel she helped make back in Blanco. We placed the panel at the Modonna Church. Pictures Gabby took tell the story. Martha still grieved when she is reminded of her loss. Her tears soon turn to smiles when she went to that evening's raffle and snack time.

We also felt blessed for our time together with Martha at NCAN as she died the following year in May, 2004.

We also left the NCAN conference on a sad note, when we learned this would be the last year Fr. Rodney and Leo (the Registrar) would be in charge of the conference. The search was on for a new director for next year's conference. Just before we went to the banquet, several awards were presented to both Fr. Rodney and Frederick. Rodney's brother and his wife, as well as Frederick's sister were present for this special event.

Gabby, Martha and I all lamented how difficult it would be not to have Rodney and Leo as our leaders. Although they both told us we would hear from them again, as of this date (September 21, 2006), we have received no word from either one of them.

Gabby and I have often said how much we miss Rodney and Frederick since we last saw them that July 2003. That would also be the last year we traveled to Chicago.

The new year 2004, began with me being interviewed by one of the NAHOF Board member, Cynthia Poindexter, Ph.d.of New York, N.Y. Cynthia was writing a research article for the

Journal of HIV/AIDS based on the interviews of six of us described as "champions" who described how we were being over age 50 and living with HIV. Cynthia sent me a draft copy as well as the final product. I thought, "Now I am part of a written research publication. Wow!"

Then, on March 16, 2004, Molly Gintry, a WE News correspondent, interviewed me. She wrote about HIV/AIDS cases are still rising among older women.

On April 23, 2004, I was co-presenter at the Austin Travis County Health and Human Services Department. The other speaker was Barrbara Joseph, who also founded an HIV organization, which provides HIV education and risk reduction in communities with special emphasis on women. She has been infected for the same amount of time as me.

From June 28 to August 13, 2004, I participated in a U.T. @ Austin Research Project – Health Promotion for Women with HIV: Phrase II – A Pilot Intervention Study. The focus of the study was to explore ways adults with HIV can enhance and maintain their health.

Then Gabby and I both were notified we were

given scholarships to attend the 17th NCAN HIV/ AIDS Ministry Conference scheduled for July 16-19,2004. We had to turn them down as we experienced unexpected home repairs. We had to use our savings to redo one of our bathrooms that collapsed.

The last event of 1994, I was interviewed and pictures taken for the World AIDS Day issue of a new Hispanic publication called RUMBO. It was written in Spanish and told how I survived 20 years living with HIV.

The year 2005 reflects only two significant events that year. The first was receipt of a certificate dated August 7, 2004 but mailed in 1995, to acknowledge my participation in the U.T. research project last summer.

The other was when I was invited to speak at the Kick-Off Dinner held Friday, April 28, 2005 sponsored by the Austin Care Alliance. Our oldest son, Roger. spoke before me. I was so touched by his words, which I chose to use as a "forward" in this book.

For many years I have been told I should write my story about how I have lived so long with HIV. When I passed the 20+ years of living and still being healthy, I decided I would. It took until early this year in March, I began writing. I am not a journalist by any means, but over the years I've written many speeches or as I call them, talks about my experiences living with my now lifetime partner called HIV.

I have learned many lessons   throughout this journey, some funny, sad, happy and sometimes wow me. All have taught me lessons I needed to learn.

I am so blessed I have the family I have: my husband is numero uno (1), and then there are our five children, (some with children, totaling 8 grandchildren) and 2 great grand-children. I also have an extended family: my two sisters, one brother, a sister-in-law, many nieces and nephews. Plus, I must include Dr. David Wright, to whom I owe so much; he is always on top of my health issues, and gave me his unlisted phone number whenever I have a real situation, which needs his immediate attention. And to all my friends here at home and all over the world, I hope this book gives everyone the real truth of what it is like living with this horrendous virus and for young people to realize how important it is to avoid getting infected; not because of the pain of endurimg the affects of the disease, but mainly because our youth are my future, our future and if reading my story prevents only one person to make the right decision, then I have accomplished my life goal.